THE QUIC EFFORTLESS SUGAR DETOX FOR YOU

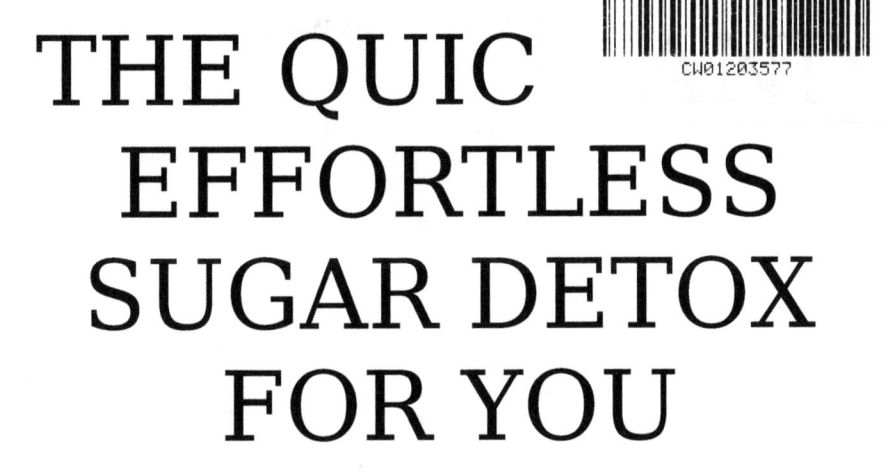

Burn Those Sugar Forever!!!

DIANA WATSON

Copyright © 2017 Diana Watson

BOOK ONE

INSULIN RESISTANCE DIET PLAN FOR TYPE 2 DIABETICS

YOUR ESSENTIAL GUIDE TO DIABETES PREVENTION AND DELICIOUS RECIPES YOU CAN ENJOY!

DIANA WATSON

TABLE OF CONTENTS

THE QUICK AND EFFORTLESS SUGAR DETOX FOR YOU
Burn Those Sugar Forever!!!
INTRODUCTION
UNDERSTAND THE RESISTANCE
INSULIN RESISTANCE DIET
LONG-TERM MANAGEMENT
DIET PLAN
RECIPES
Chapter 1: Diabetes and A Realistic Diet Plan

VIP Subscriber List

Hi Dear Reader, this is Diana! If you like my book and you want to receive the latest tips and tricks on cooking, weight-loss, cookbook recipes and more, do subscribe to my mailing list in the link here! I will then be able to send you the most up-to-date information about my upcoming books and promotions as well! Thank you for supporting my work and happy reading!

INTRODUCTION

Congratulations on purchasing your personal copy of *Insulin Resistance Diet Plan for Type 2 Diabetics.* Thank you for doing so.

If you find you are being warned by your doctor that you are at high risk of developing diabetes, or that you have insulin resistance, you're not alone. In fact, it's believed that the number of diabetics is going to double from around 190 million to 325 million within the next couple of decades. A study performed in 2002 found that 32.2% of the population in the US are insulin resistant.

Knowing how insulin resistance works on a cellular level helps people know the best ways to treat and prevent type 2 diabetes. Individuals who suffer from diabetes mellitus and obese people are often insulin resistant. Many studies have discovered that an insulin resistance diet and exercise can alter the pathways and slow down the onset of insulin resistance.

It's safe to say that if we look at ways to change our habits, and pay attention to what we do, we can make some improvements to our life. An insulin resistance diet can help you to lose weight and will turn regulate your blood glucose and insulin levels so that your chances of developing diabetes are lowered.

It's possible that insulin resistance is the leading cause of many of today's chronic diseases. These diseases are collectively killing over a million people each year. The good thing is that it can easily be improved with some simple changed in your eating, lifestyle, and exercise habits. Preventing the chance of insulin resistance is probably the best thing you can do to make sure you live a long, healthy life. There are plenty of books on this subject on the market, thanks again for choosing this one! Every effort was made to ensure it is full of as much useful information as possible. Please enjoy!

Congratulations on downloading your personal copy of *Insulin Resistance Diet Plan for Type 2 Diabetics*. Thank you for doing so.

UNDERSTAND THE RESISTANCE

There are times when our cells quit responding to our insulin. When this happens, you are likely suffering from insulin resistance. Your cells become resistant to insulin. When your body becomes resistant, your pancreas will respond by producing more insulin to try and reduce your blood sugar levels. When this happens you develop hyperinsulinemia, which is when the blood contains high levels of insulin. Let's make this a little easier, let's look at the separate parts of insulin resistance.

Metabolism

Metabolism is probably one of the most misunderstood processes that the body goes through. Your metabolism works as a collection of chemical reactions that happens in your cells to help you convert food into energy. As you are reading this, a thousand metabolic reactions are happening. There are two main metabolic channels.

- Catabolism is the process your body goes through when breaking down you food components, as in fats, proteins, and carbs, into simpler parts, which are then used for energy. To better understand it, look at it as if it is your destructive metabolism. Your cells break down fats and carbs to release their energy; this ensures that your body can fuel an anabolic reaction.

- Anabolism is the contrastive metabolism which works to build and store energy. When your cells perform an anabolic process, it helps to grow new cells and to maintain your body tissues, and it also helps to store energy that you can use later.

- The nervous and hormone systems control

these processes. When you look at how many calories you should consume in a day, you have to check your body's total energy expenditure. What you eat, how much you move, how you rest, and how well your tissues and cells recuperate will all go into figuring out your total energy expenditure.

- Your metabolism is made up of three main components:

1. Basal metabolic rate – this how many calories you body can burn while at rest, and also contributes to 50 to 80 percent of the amount of energy you body uses.

2. How much energy is used during activity – this is how many calories your body burns when you are active. This takes up 20% of your total expenditure.

3. Warming effects of your food – this is how

many calories you use when you eat, digest, and metabolize your food.

4. Insulin

5. Insulin is a hormone that the pancreas produces and releases into your blood. Insulin help to keep your blood sugar at a reasonable level by promoting cell growth and division, protein and lipid metabolism, regulating carbohydrates, and glucose uptake. Insulin helps your cells absorb glucose to use for energy.

6. After you eat, and your blood sugar levels rise, insulin is released. The glucose and insulin travel throughout your blood to your cells. It helps to stimulate the muscle tissue and liver; helps liver, fat, and muscle cells to absorb glucose; and lowers glucose levels by reducing the glucose production in your liver.

7. People who suffer from type 1 or type 2 diabetes may have to take insulin shot to help their bodies metabolize glucose correctly. Type 1 diabetic's pancreas doesn't make insulin, and the beta cells have been destroyed. There's typically no chance of preventing type 1, and most of the time a person is born with it. Type 2 diabetic's pancreas still make insulin, but the body doesn't respond to it.

8. Symptoms

9. If you go to the doctor, they will likely test your fasting insulin levels. If you have high levels, then chances are you are insulin resistant. You can also do an oral glucose tolerance test. This is where you will be given a dose of glucose, and they will check your blood sugar levels for the next few hours.

10. People who are obese or overweight, and people with a lot of fat in the mid-section, are at a greater risk of being insulin resistant. Acanthosis nigrans, a skin condition characterized by dark spots on the skin, can be a symptom of insulin resistance. Also, if you have low HDL and high triglycerides, then your chances are higher as well.

11. For the most part, insulin resistance and pre-diabetes have no significant symptoms. They main way to find out if you have either one is to get tested by your doctor. Now, you're probably wondering how to know if you should be tested. Here are some reasons why you should:

- Body Mass Index over 25
- Over age 45
- Have CVD

- Physically inactive

- Parent or sibling with diabetes

- Family background of Pacific Islander American, Hispanic/Latino, Asian American, Native American, Alaska Native, or African American

- Had a baby that weighed more than 9 pounds

- Diagnoses of gestational diabetes

- High blood pressure – 140/90 or higher

- HDL below 35 or triglyceride above 250

- Have polycystic ovary syndrome

- If your tests come back as normal, be sure to be retested every three years, at least. But, you don't have to wait until you get positive test results to start changing your life. In fact, if you have any of the risk factors, even if it's just a family history, you start changing now, and you may never have to hear that diagnoses.

-
- ## INSULIN RESISTANCE DIET
- Years of research has found that excess weight is the primary cause of insulin resistance. This means that weight loss can help you body better respond to insulin. Studies performed by the Diabetes Prevention Program have found that people who are pre-diabetic and insulin resistance can prevent or slow down the development of diabetes by fixing their diet.

- **Guidelines**

- Here are the main seven ways you go start to develop an insulin resistance diet:

1. Reduce Carbohydrate Intake

2. Studies that have been published in *Diabetes, Metabolic Syndrome and Obesity* suggest that controlling the number of carbohydrates you

eat is essential in controlling your glycemic index. You can count all carbs you eat, but it's best if you make sure you consume your carbs from dairy products, legumes, whole grains, fruits, and veggies.

3. Stay Away From Sweetened Beverages

4. All sugars will raise your blood sugar levels, but the American Diabetes Association has now advised, specifically, to avoid sugar-sweetened drinks. This includes iced tea, fruit drinks, soft drinks, and vitamin or energy water drinks that have artificial sweeteners, concentrates, high fructose corn syrup, or sucrose.

5. Consume More Fiber

6. Glycemia is improved in people who consume more than 50 grams of fiber each day. Large prospective cohort studies have shown that

whole grain consumption is associated with a lower risk of type 2 diabetes.

7. Consume Healthy Fats

8. Studies have shown that fatty acids are more important than total fat. People who suffer from insulin resistance should consume unsaturated fats instead of trans fatty acids or saturated fats.

9. Consume Plenty of Protein

10. *International Journal of Vitamin and Nutrition Research* published a study in 2011 that discovered people who were on a diet to treat obesity had better results when they consumed more protein.

11. Consume Dairy

12. More and more studies are finding that dairy consumption is linked to a reduced risk of type 2 diabetes.

13. Watch Your Portions

14. Losing weight is key in reducing your risk for diabetes. One great way to do that controls your portion sizes. It's best to eat more small meals instead of three large meals.

15. Bad Foods

16. When you start the insulin resistance diet, there are certain foods that you need to avoid, or at least reduce your intake of. Here are some of the foods that you need to watch out for.

- Red meat – contains lots of saturated fats that can exacerbate the problems

- Certain cheeses – cheese that is high in fat will cause more problems

- Fried food – this is a bad dietary choice no matter what diet you're on

- Grains – processed or refined carbs can lead

higher insulin levels

- Potatoes – these foods turn into sugar in your system
- Pumpkin – these are just like potatoes
- Carrots – these aren't entirely bad for you, just limit your intake because they are high in sugar
- Doughnuts – these are full insulin raising ingredients
- Alcohol – these turn straight to sugar when you drink them
- **Good Foods**
- Now that you know the main foods you should stay away from, here are the foods you should consume.
- Broccoli, Spinach, Collard greens – these, as well as most other leafy greens, are a great

source of magnesium, zinc, vitamin E, C, and A

- Broccoli sprouts

- Swiss Chard, Romaine Lettuce, Arugula, Green Cabbage, and Kale – these also contain high amounts of nutrients

- Blueberries – contain anthocyanins which simulate the release of adiponectin which helps regular blood sugar

- Indian gooseberry – these can regulate blood sugar and reduce hyperglycemia

- Walnuts – any nut is great food for an insulin resistance diet

- These are just a few of some of the foods you should consume. Many other foods have the same properties as the ones on this list, as well as a few other types of benefits.

-
-

-
- **LONG-TERM MANAGEMENT**
- Once you have started a diet, the hardest thing is sticking with it. The good thing about this diet is that it isn't anything drastic, and you can quickly change your diet with a few tweaks. To ensure that you have lasting results, let's look at some of the best ways to maintain.
- Be sure to keep up regular exercise. Exercise can help lower your blood sugar, reduce body fat, and help you lose weight. Your cells will also become more insulin sensitive as well. You don't have to do anything spectacular either. Any movement will help you; gardening, running, swimming, walking, or dancing all count for exercise.
- Remember that weight loss isn't going to be linear. You may start dropping pounds when

you first start, but you will eventually hit a plateau. You have to be proactive with your diet. When you notice you are hitting a plateau, start to make little changes to push past it.

- Try to pay attention to when you eat. If you notice that you eat when you are stress, upset, sad, bored, lonely, or low on energy take note of it. Look for other ways to move past those emotions to prevent emotional eating.
- Find some cheerleaders. I don't mean paying people to follow you around all day cheering, that would get annoying. I mean you should find a support system. The main reason why diet programs like Jenny Craig and Weight Watchers works are because of the meeting and people to talk to. There's no need to pay big bucks for this thought. You can get your family and friends to help you out, and you can

probably find a Facebook group to help you out.

- **Side Effects**
- With any diet, you will experience some side effects. These side effects will either be longer-term or short-term. Let's look at some side effects that you may experience when you begin the insulin resistance diet.
- Short-term:
    - Cravings – this is normal when you start to change your diet. Your body becomes freaked out when you start to eat healthier foods and reduce the snack foods that you're used to eating. Keep reminding yourself why you're doing this. The cravings will eventually pass.
    - Headaches – this is because your body has become addicted to the processed foods you're used to eating. You're going

to withdrawals. Once you get all the bad food out of your system, the headaches will stop.

- o Lower energy – this is another symptom you will have because of withdrawals. Your energy levels will drop. Your body is doing a lot of work when you start eating healthier, so be patient with it.

- Long-term:

    - o Weight loss – this is probably the best thing that will happen to you on this diet. Weight loss will help to improve all of your health problems.

    - o Less hunger and cravings – you may start out having more cravings, but once that phase passes, you won't be bothered with the hunger and cravings like you used to be.

- Lower blood pressure – a diet that is low in sugar and trans and saturated fats, your blood pressure will lower. This reduces your risk of heart disease, heart attack, stroke, and several other health problems.

- More energy – getting rid of high glycemic index foods will give bursts of energy that you have never had. Plus, you will no longer have the rollercoaster effect from your blood sugar highs and lows.

- Better mood and concentration – with your old diet, you probably had mood boosts followed by a sudden plummet. With the insulin resistance diet, you will keep a more steady mood and concentration throughout the day.

- Better immune system – since you won't be consuming as many inflammatory and allergenic foods you will be able to improve your overall immune system and health.
- Increased digestion – with this diet you will reduce your intake of sugar, dairy, and gluten. These foods are the most common foods to cause digestive problems. Since you won't be consuming as many of these foods, your digestive system will work better. You will also increase your fiber intake, so this will aid your gastrointestinal tract as well.
- As you can see, the long-term side effects are better than the short-term side effects; there are also more long-term effects. It's easy to see the good outweighs the bad. It's a no brainer that

this is an easy and simple diet to follow.

-
-
-
-

-
- ## DIET PLAN
- To help get you started, here is a 5-day meal plan. All of the recipes will follow in the next chapter.
- <u>Day One</u>
- Breakfast: Basil and Tomato Frittata
- Frittatas are the perfect breakfast to help use up leftovers. Pair this with a slice of whole grain toast and fruit.
- Lunch: Carrot and Butternut Squash Soup
- You'll never go back to canned soups after you try this.
- Dinner: Grilled Shrimp Skewers
- This is a quick meal because shrimp only takes a few minutes to cook.

- <u>Day Two</u>
- Breakfast: Pecan, Carrot, and Banana Muffins
- This is a meal you can serve to your friends, and nobody will ever know that they are healthy. It's the perfect guilt-free treat.
- Lunch: Lemony Hummus
- Creating your hummus is a great meal. You have control over its flavor and salt levels.
- Dinner: Chicken Tortilla Soup
- This is perfect if you have some leftover chicken. This spicy soup will satisfy everyone.
- <u>Day Three</u>
- Breakfast: Dried Fruit, Seeds, and Nuts

Granola

- This is great to mix up a large amount on the weekend and portion it out for the following week.
- There is a high carb content because of the dried fruit, but you can easily fix that by reducing the fruit or leaving it out entirely.
- Lunch: Quinoa Tabbouleh Salad
- Quinoa is the perfect food because not only is it gluten-free, but it's also considered a protein. This is a delicious meal for meat-eaters and vegetarians.
- Dinner: Rice and Beef Stuffed Peppers
- These little peppers look sophisticated, but the entire family will love eating them up.

- <u>Day Four</u>
- Breakfast: Goat Cheese and Veggie Scramble
- This is the perfect savory breakfast. With the onions, tomatoes, peppers, eggs, and cheese you have the perfect well-rounded meal.
- Lunch: Curried Chicken Salad
- The Greek yogurt and mayo adds creaminess to the sandwich that you won't get anywhere else.
- Dinner: Jamaican Pork Tenderloin with Beans
- This is a quick summertime meal that everybody will love. Serve alongside some pilaf or brown rice.
- <u>Day Five</u>

- Breakfast: Superfood Smoothie
- This four ingredient smoothie is quick to whip up and won't run you late.
- Lunch: Tomato and Spinach Pasta
- This dish is perfect for lunch or dinner. Make a double portion so you can have some later in the week.
- Dinner: Grilled Turkey Burgers
- It should never be said that you can't have a tasty and healthy burger. Fix some sweet potato fries to complete this meal.

- RECIPES
- **Sides & Extras**
- **Salsa**
- Ingredients:
- Salt
- 1 tbsp olive oil
- ½ lime
- 1 minced garlic clove
- 1/3 c coriander, chopped
- 1 jalapeno, chopped
- 1 onion, chopped
- 2 tomatoes, chopped
- Instructions:
- Mix everything together. Add salt to your taste. Allow refrigerating for 30 minutes.

- **Oven-Roasted Tomatoes**
- Ingredients:
- salt
- 1 tbsp oil
- 4 thyme sprigs
- 1-pint cherry tomatoes, halved
- Instructions:
- The oven should be at 320. Place the tomatoes on a prepared baking sheet. Top with salt and thyme and drizzle with oil. Cook for 45 minutes.

- **Zucchini Chips**
- Ingredients:
- salt
- 1 tbsp olive oil
- 4 zucchini, sliced
- Instructions:
- Place the zucchini slices on a prepared baking sheet. Top with oil and salt.
- Cook for 30 minutes at 320 until they brown.

-
- **Breakfast**
- **Basil and Tomato Frittata**
- Ingredients:
- ½ c Italian cheese, reduced-fat
- ¼ tsp pepper
- ¼ tsp salt
- 8 egg whites
- ¼ c basil, sliced
- 2 plum tomatoes
- 1 minced garlic clove
- 2 tsp EVOO
- ¼ c onion, chopped
- Instructions:
- Cook the onion in a hot skillet until it has become tender. Mix the garlic until fragrant.

Stir in the tomato and cook until all the liquid is absorbed. Add in the basil.

- Mix the pepper, salt, and eggs. Pour into the skillet over the veggies, and top with cheese. Slide the skillet into an oven that is set to broil. Cook until the eggs are set.

- **Pecan, Carrot, and Banana Muffin**
- Ingredients:
- ¼ c pecans, chopped
- 1 tsp vanilla
- ½ c banana, mashed
- ¾ c carrot, shredded
- 1/3 c yogurt, sugar-free
- 1 egg
- 1/3 c brown sugar
- ¼ c canola oil
- ½ tsp salt
- ¼ tsp baking soda
- 1 tsp cinnamon
- 1 tsp baking powder
- 1 c whole wheat flour

- Instructions:

- Mix the flour, baking powder, cinnamon, baking soda, and salt together.

- Mix all the other ingredients, except for the nuts. Once combine, mix into the flour mixture. Gently fold in the pecans.

- Pour into a prepared 6-cup muffin tin. In should bake for 22 minutes at 375.

- **Homemade Granola**
- Ingredients:
- ½ c brown sugar
- 1 ½ tsp salt
- ¼ c maple syrup
- ¾ c honey
- 1 c oil
- 2 tsp vanilla
- ½ c dried apricots
- ½ c sultans
- ½ c dried cranberries
- ½ c coconut flakes
- 1 c cashews
- 1 c walnuts
- ½ c flaked almonds
- 1 c pecans, chopped
- ½ c pepitas
- 1 c sunflower seeds
- 8 c rolled oats

- Directions:
- The oven should be at 325. Mix the nuts, coconut, and oats. In a pot mix the brown sugar, vanilla, sugar, oil, honey, maple syrup and allow to boil. Let it cook for five minutes until thick. Pour the sugar mixture over the nuts and quickly stir together.
- Place the mixture on baking sheets lined with foil. Cook for 10 minutes. Remove and mix up the mixture. Bake for another 10 minutes. Once it's browned, mix in the dried fruits. Once cool, seal in a bowl or bag.
-

- **Goat Cheese and Veggie Scramble**
- Ingredients:
- ¼ c goat cheese
- ¼ tsp pepper
- ¼ tsp salt
- 1 c egg substitute
- ½ c tomato, chopped
- 2 tsp olive oil
- ¼ c onion, chopped
- ¼ c bell pepper, chopped
- Instructions:
- Cook the pepper and onion until soft. Mix in the tomato and cook until liquid is absorbed. Turn down the heat and add in the egg substitute, pepper, and salt. Scramble the egg until cooked through. Top with goat cheese.

-
- **Superfood Smoothie**
- Instructions:
- 1 banana
- 2 c spinach
- 1 c blueberries, frozen
- 1 c almond milk
- Instructions:
- Place everything in your blender and mix until smooth.

-
- **Lunch**
- **Carrot and Butternut Squash Soup**
- ¼ c half-and-half, fat-free
- ¼ tsp nutmeg
- ¼ tsp pepper
- 2 14 ½ -oz can chicken broth, reduced-sodium
- ¾ c leeks, sliced
- 2 c carrots, sliced
- 3 c butternut squash, diced
- 1 tbsp butter
- Instructions:
- Melt the butter in a large pot. Place the leek, carrot, and squash in the hot pot. Put on the lid, and allow to cook for about eight minutes. Pour in the broth. Allow everything to come to

boil. Turn down the heat to a simmer. Place the lid on the pot and let cook for 25 minutes. The veggies should be tender.

- With an immersion blender, mix the soup to the consistency that you like. Season with the nutmeg and the pepper. Bring everything back to a boil and stir in the half-and-half.

-

- **Lemony Hummus**
- Ingredients:
- ¼ c water
- 1 tbsp EVOO
- ¼ tsp cumin
- ¼ tsp pepper
- ½ tsp salt
- 1 clove garlic, chopped
- 1 ½ tbsp tahini
- ¼ c lemon juice
- 15-oz chickpeas, drained
- Directions:
- Add everything except for the water and oil in a food processor. Mix until combine. Add the oil and water and continue mixing until smooth. Add extra water if you need to.

- **Quinoa Tabbouleh**
- Ingredients:
- 2 scallions, sliced
- ½ c mint, chopped
- 2/3 c parsley
- 1-pint cherry tomatoes
- 1 large cucumber
- pepper
- ½ c EVOO
- 1 minced garlic clove
- 2 tbsp lemon juice
- ½ tsp salt
- 1 c quinoa, rinsed
- Instructions:
- Cook the quinoa in salted water. As the quinoa cooks, mix the garlic and lemon juice. Slowly

whisk in the EVOO, and then sprinkle with pepper and salt to your taste.

- Allow the quinoa to cool completely. Toss with the dressing and then mix in the remaining ingredients. Add extra pepper and salt if needed.

- **Curried Chicken Salad**
- Ingredients:
- 4 whole wheat pita rounds
- 2 c mixed greens
- 1 c green grapes
- ¼ tsp pepper
- ¼ tsp salt
- 1 tsp curry powder
- 3 tbsp mayo, reduced-fat
- ½ c Greek yogurt, nonfat
- ¼ c slivered almonds
- 1 ¼-lb chicken, shredded
- Instructions:
- Mix all of the ingredients except for the greens and pitas. Divide the chicken mixture into each pita. Top each with some greens.

-
- **Tomato and Spinach Pasta**
- Instructions:
- 3 tbsp parmesan, grated
- 1 tbsp balsamic vinegar
- ¼ tsp pepper
- 2 minced garlic cloves
- 1 c grape tomatoes
- 8 c spinach
- 2 tbsp olive oil
- 8-oz whole-wheat spaghetti
- Instructions:
- Cook the spaghetti the way the package says to, but without the salt. Drain.
- As the pasta cooks, sauté the spinach until it wilts. Stir in the tomatoes and cook for about three minutes. Mix in the garlic.

- Toss the pasta with the veggies and all the other ingredients.

-
- **Dinner**
- **Grilled Shrimp Skewers**
- Ingredients:
- 9 skewers, soaked
- 1 lb cleaned shrimp
- 2 scallions, minced
- ¼ tsp pepper
- ½ tsp salt
- ¼ tsp red pepper flakes
- 1 medium lemon, zest, and juice
- 2 minced garlic cloves
- 1 ½ tbsp olive oil
- Instructions:
- Prepare your grill.
- Mix the scallions, pepper, salt, pepper flakes,

lemon juice and zest, garlic, and oil.

- Place the shrimp in the mixture and coat. Allow to marinate in the refrigerate for 30 minutes.

- Place the shrimp evenly among the skewers. Get rid on any remaining marinade.

- Grill them shrimp until pink and firm, around two to three minutes.

-

- **Chicken Tortilla Soup**
- Ingredients:
- 1 c tortilla chips
- 2 minced garlic cloves
- 1 c chicken broth, reduced-sodium
- 2 c stir-fry veggies
- 2 c chicken, shredded
- 2 ½ c water
- 1 14 ½-oz can stewed tomatoes, Mexican-style
- Directions:
- In a crock pot, mix the garlic, broth, veggies, chicken, water, and tomatoes.
- Cook for six and a half hours on low.
- Top with chips.

- **Rice and Beef Stuffed Peppers**
- Ingredients:
- 1 tbsp parsley, divided
- ½ tsp pepper
- 2 tsp salt
- 4 minced garlic cloves
- ½ c tomato sauce
- ¼ c parsley
- ½ c Parmigiano-Reggiano, shredded
- 1 ½ c rice, cooked
- 1 ½ lb ground beef
- ¼ tsp red pepper flakes
- 1 c beef broth
- ½ onion, sliced
- 2 ½ c tomato sauce
- 6 bell peppers
- Instructions:
- The oven should be at 375. Cut the tops off the peppers and clean out the insides. Poke a few

small holes in the bottom of each.

- Place 2 ½ cups tomato sauce in a casserole dish. Place in the pepper flakes, broth, and onion. Set the peppers upright in the mixture.
- Mix the pepper, salt, garlic, 2 tbsp tomato sauce, ¼ c parsley, cheese, rice, and beef. Divide the mixture between the peppers. Add a tablespoon of tomato sauce on top of each and lay the pepper tops back on. Top dish with parchment paper and then tin foil. Place the dish on a baking sheet.
- Cook for an hour. They should be starting to feel soft. Take off the foil and parchment and cook for an addition 25 minutes.
-

-
- **Jamaican Pork Tenderloin**
- Ingredients:
- ½ tsp pepper
- ¼ tsp salt
- 1 tbsp lemon juice
- 1 tsp lemon zest
- 1 tbsp EVOO
- 1 lb green beans
- 3 c water
- 2 tbsp Creole mustard
- ¼ c grape jelly
- 2 tsp Jerk seasoning
- ¼ c orange juice, divided
- ¾ lb pork tenderloin
- Instructions:
- Mix the pepper, salt, lemon juice and zest, EVOO and water. Bring everything to a boil and add in the beans.
- As the beans cook, mix the mustard, jelly, jerk

seasoning, and half the orange juice. Cover the tenderloin. The oven should be set and 350. Place the tenderloin in a casserole dish and pour in the rest of the orange juice. Bake for 45 minutes.

-

- **Grilled Turkey Burgers**
- Ingredients:
- 4 whole-wheat buns
- ½ tsp curry
- ¼ c Dijon
- 12-oz ground turkey
- 1/8 tsp pepper
- ¼ tsp garlic salt
- ¼ tsp Italian seasoning
- 2 tbsp milk, fat-free
- 2 tbsp bread crumbs
- ¼ c green onions, sliced
- ½ c carrot, shredded
- Instructions:
- Mix the ground turkey with the seasonings, bread crumbs, and veggies. Form the meat mixture into four patties.
- Prepare your grill, and cook the patties until done.

- Mix the mustard and curry powder and spread onto the buns. Add the burgers to the buns. Top with tomato and lettuce if desired.

-
- **Dessert**
- **Blueberries and Yogurt**
- Ingredients:
- 1/3 c Greek yogurt
- 10 blueberries
- Instructions:
- Top the yogurt with the blueberries and enjoy.
-

-
- **Raspberry Sorbet**
- Ingredients:
- lemon juice
- 1 c raspberries
- Instructions:
- Place the ingredients in a food processor and mix until smooth. Place in an airtight container and freeze.
-

•

•

•

•

•

•

•

•

•

•

BOOK TWO

THE SUPREME METABOLISM DIET

Turbo Boost Your Metabolism To

An Amazing Body

-
- DIANA WATSON

- Copyright © 2017 Diana Watson
- All rights reserved.

TABLE OF CONTENTS

- THE QUICK AND EFFORTLESS SUGAR DETOX FOR YOU
- *Burn Those Sugar Forever!!!*
- INTRODUCTION
- UNDERSTAND THE RESISTANCE
- INSULIN RESISTANCE DIET
- LONG-TERM MANAGEMENT
- DIET PLAN
- RECIPES
- THE SUPREME METABOLISM DIET
- *Turbo Boost Your Metabolism To An Amazing Body*

- WHAT IS METABOLISM?
- PHASE 1
  - ....BREAKFAST
  - ....CINNAMON APPLE QUINOA
  - ....LUNCH
  - ....MASHED CHICKPEA SALAD
  - ....DINNER
  - ......SLOW COOKER SPAGHETTI AND MEATBALLS
- PHASE 2
  - ....BREAKFAST
  - ....KOREAN ROLLED OMELETTE
  - ....LUNCH

- • • MARINATED TOFU WITH PEPPERS AND ONIONS
- • DINNER
- • • • • • • • • ROAST BEEF AND VEGETABLES
- PHASE 3
- • BREAKFAST
- • • • • • • • • BERRY COBBLER WITH QUINOA
- • LUNCH
- • • • • • • • • • • • • • ITALIAN TUNA SALAD
- • DINNER
- • • • • • • SHEET PAN STEAK AND VEGGIES
- DOS AND DON'TS
- CONCLUSION

Chapter 1: Diabetes and A Realistic Diet Plan

INTRODUCTION

Congratulations on purchasing your personal copy of *The Supreme Metabolism Diet..* Thank you for doing so.

The following chapters will provide with information and recipes so that you can get started on the Fast Metabolism Diet today.

- There are plenty of books on this subject on the market, thanks again for choosing this one! Every effort was made to ensure it is full of as much useful information as possible. Please enjoy!

- Congratulations on purchasing your personal copy of *Fast Metabolism Diet Cookbook*. Thank you for doing so.

-

-

WHAT IS METABOLISM?

Metabolism is typically used when we are describing different chemical reactions that help to maintain healthy organisms and cells. There are two types of metabolism:

- Anabolism: the synthesis of the compounds that the cell need.

- Catabolism: the breaking down of the molecules to get energy.

- Metabolism is closely linked to a person's nutrition and how they use their available nutrients. Bioenergetics tells us how our metabolic or biochemical paths for our cells use energy. Forming energy is a vital component in metabolism.

- Good nutrition is the key to metabolism. Metabolism requires nutrients so they can break down to produce energy. This energy is needed to make new nucleic acids, proteins, etc.

- Diets need nutrients like sulfur, phosphorus, nitrogen, oxygen, hydrogen, carbon, and 20 other inorganic elements. These elements are received from proteins, lipids, and carbohydrates. Water, minerals, and vitamins are necessary.

- Your body gets carbs in three different ways from food: sugar, cellulose, and starch. Sugars and starches form essential sources of energy for us humans.

- Body tissues need glucose for everyday

activities. Sugars and carbs give off glucose by metabolism or digestion.

- Most people's diet is half carbs. These carbs typically come from macaroni, pasta, potatoes, bread, wheat, rice, etc.

- The tissue builders of the body are proteins. Proteins are found in every cell of the human body. Proteins help with enzymes that carry out needed reactions, hemoglobin formation to carry the oxygen, functions, cell structure, and many other functions within the body. Proteins are needed to supply nitrogen for DNA, producing energy, and RNA genetic material.

- Protein is necessary for nutrition since they have amino acids. The human body can't synthesize eight of these, and they are amino acids that are essential to us.

- These amino acids are:

- Threonine
- Valine
- Phenylalanine
- Isoleucine
- Leucine
- Methionine
- Tryptophan
- Lysine
- Foods that have the best quality of protein are grains, vegetables, meats, soybeans, milk, and eggs.
- Fats are a more condensed form of energy. They make twice the amount of energy as proteins or carbs.
- These are the functions of fats:
- Provide a reserve for energy.
- Help to absorb fat soluble vitamins.

- Forms a protection insulation and cushion around vital organs.
- Helps to form a cellular structure.
- The fatty acids that are required include unsaturated acids, such as arachidonic, linolenic, and linoleic acids. These are needed in the diet. Cholesterol and saturated fats have been associated with heart disease and arteriosclerosis.
- Minerals found in food don't give you energy, but they do play a role in your bodies pathways and are important regulators. There are more than 50 elements that can be found in the body. Only 25 have been deemed essential so far. Deficiency in these could produce specific symptoms.
- These are the essential minerals:
- Iodine

- Fluorine
- Magnesium
- Zinc
- Manganese
- Cobalt
- Copper
- Chloride ions
- Potassium
- Sodium
- Iron
- Phosphorus
- Calcium
- Vitamins are known as organic compounds that the human body is unable to synthesize by itself, so they need to be found within your diet. These are the most important vitamins in metabolism:

- Pantothenic Acid

- Nicotinic acid or Niacin

- B2 or riboflavin

- Vitamin A

- Metabolism's chemical reactions are grouped within your metabolic pathways. This gives the chemicals that come from your nutrition to be changed through several different steps along with another chemical. This is done with a series of enzymes.

- Enzymes are important for your metabolism because they give organisms the ability to achieve the reactions that they need for energy. These also work along with the others that release energy. Enzymes are basically catalysts that let these reactions happen efficiently and quickly.

-

-
- # PHASE 1

- While on this diet you will rotate the way you eat between three phases:
- Phase One – Monday and Tuesday:
- Phase Two – Wednesday and Thursday:
- Phase Three – Friday, Saturday, and Sunday:
- Repeat this for four weeks.
- Every phase focuses on different healthy, whole foods to help reduce your liver stress, calm your adrenal glands, and feed your thyroid. Now, let's look at phase one and some recipes to get you started.
- Phase One – low-fat, moderate-protein, high-glycemic
- One of the main things that phase one will help you with is by regulating your adrenal

glands. The adrenal glands secrete stress hormones, which is only useful when you are in immediate danger. When you aren't in danger, all it will do for you is raise your cortisol level, which causes weight gain.

- In phase one, you will eat higher glycemic fruits because they stimulate your pituitary gland, which is your pleasure center. This releases endorphins which will reduce anxiety and stress.
- In phase one you will also need to do some cardio, this will help to reduce cortisol levels even more.
- BREAKFAST
- CINNAMON APPLE QUINOA
- Serves: 2
- Ingredients:
- Honey

- 2 tsp cinnamon
- 2 large apples
- 1 ½ c water
- ½ c quinoa
- Instructions:
- Prepare the apples by coring and peeling. Chop the prepared apples into small pieces.
- Place the apples, quinoa, and water into a pot. Allow the mixture to come to a boil. Place the lid on the pot and turn the heat down to a simmer. Let cook for 20 to 25 minutes. The apples should be soft, and the quinoa should have absorbed all the water.
- Mix in the cinnamon and divide between two bowls.
- Drizzle the top with some more cinnamon and honey.
- LUNCH
- MASHED CHICKPEA SALAD

- Serves: 2
- Ingredients:
- Pepper and salt to your taste
- 1 ½ tbsp sunflower seeds
- ½ lemon, juiced
- ½ tsp garlic, minced
- 3 tbsp Dijon
- 2 tbsp cilantro
- ½ c kale, chopped
- ¼ c red onion, chopped
- 1/3 of an apple, chopped
- 2 celery stalks, chopped
- 15-oz chickpeas, rinsed and drained
- 1 carrot, shredded
- Instructions:
- Shred your carrot in a food processor and

place in a large bowl.

- Place the chickpeas in the processor and pulse a couple of times until well blended, but a little chunky. If you want, you can just use a potato masher.
- Place chickpeas and the rest of the ingredients in the bowl with the carrot. Mix everything together and add pepper and salt to your taste.
- DINNER
- SLOW COOKER SPAGHETTI AND MEATBALLS
- Serves: 6
- Ingredients:
- Meatballs:
- ½ tsp pepper
- 1 tsp salt

- ½ c breadcrumbs
- 2 eggs
- 1 ½ tsp oregano
- ¼ c parsley, minced
- 3 minced garlic
- ½ onion, grated
- 1 ½ lb lean ground beef
- Sauce:
- 16-oz whole wheat spaghetti drained and cooked
- 4 basil leaves, sliced
- 14-oz crushed tomatoes
- 28-oz crushed tomatoes
- ½ tsp pepper
- ½ tsp salt
- ½ tsp sugar

- 4-oz tomato paste

- 1 tsp oregano

- 1 onion, chopped

- 3 minced garlic cloves

- 1 tbsp olive oil

- Instructions:

- Meatballs:

- Your oven should be at 350. Spray a baking sheet with nonstick spray.

- Mix the pepper, salt, breadcrumbs, eggs, oregano, parsley, garlic, onion, and beef together.

- For the meat mixture into balls. Place them on the baking sheet, evenly spaced.

- Bake until they are almost cooked, about 12 to 15 minutes. Transfer your meatballs to your slow cookers and scrape off bits of fat from the bottom of the meatballs.

- Sauce:

- Place the oil in a pan and heat. Place in the garlic and cook for a few seconds.

- Mix in the oregano and onion. Cooking for about three minutes, the onions should be soft.

- Stir in the pepper, salt, sugar, and tomato paste and cook another two minutes.

- Mix in the basil and crushed tomatoes. Pour the mixture over the meatballs in your cooker.

- Cook for five hours at low. Serve the mixture over your cooked spaghetti.

-

-

-
- ## PHASE 2

- Phase 2 – low-fat, low-carb, high-veggie, high-protein

- Lean proteins provide the ingredients that create amino acids within the body. Alkaline vegetables provide enzymes and phytonutrients that break down the proteins. The amino acids are converted into muscle.

- Muscles are insatiable. They need lots of fuel. The more muscle you have, the more fat you are going to burn. Muscle works for you. It burns fat that has been stored as fuel to help melt away stubborn fat. More muscle means higher metabolic rate. Muscle-building is about weight training. You can use your body weight, hand weight, weight machines, or dumbbells.

- When you eat lean proteins such as chicken, fish, turkey, bison, and beef, the stomach will start to secrete pepsinogen that converts into the enzyme pepsin. This pepsin will start breaking down the protein into amino acids.

- This phase isn't all about eating protein. If you were to eat nothing but protein, your body's pH balance would begin to be far too acidic and you will start to feel ill. To balance out this protein, you will be eating a lot of alkalizing vegetables like collard greens, cucumbers, spinach, kale, broccoli, and cabbage. These vegetables give the body more alkaline thus bringing the body's pH into balance.

- The other good things happening in this phase is all the vitamin C that you are consuming is strengthening the adrenal glands, and we know that strong adrenal glands react less to stress.

- Iodine and taurine in the vegetables will nourish the thyroid thus prepping it to release the fat-burning hormones that will be coming in the next phase.
- BREAKFAST
- KOREAN ROLLED OMELETTE
- Serves: 1
- Ingredients:
- Roasted seaweed
- 2 pinches salt
- 3 eggs
- ½ tsp butter
- Instructions:
- Whisk the eggs together with some salt.
- Butter a pan lightly.
- Heat the pan and pour in the whisked eggs.
- Let them cook until they are almost set, then place a sheet of seaweed on top.
- Take a spatula and lift an edge of the egg over

the seaweed. Continue to roll the egg over the seaweed. Allow it to cool slightly and then slice into one-inch pieces.

- LUNCH
- MARINATED TOFU WITH PEPPERS AND ONIONS
- Serves: 4
- Ingredients:
- 3 red bell peppers, seeded and sliced
- 1 red onion, sliced into ¼-inch thick rounds
- 1 tbsp honey
- 4 tbsp EVOO, divided
- 1 lb block medium tofu, sliced into ½-inch slices
- Pepper and salt
- ¾ tsp paprika, divided
- 3 ½ tsp cumin, divided

- ¼ c garlic, minced
- 2/3 c lime juice
- ¾ c cilantro, chopped
- Instructions:
- Your oven should be at 450. Place foil onto a baking sheet. Mix ½ teaspoon paprika, 3 teaspoon cumin, garlic, lime juice, and ¼ cup cilantro together. Sprinkle with pepper and salt. Pour half of the marinade into a baggie. Place in the tofu. Seal the bag and shake so everything is coated. Allow to marinate at room temp for ten to fifteen minutes, flip over occasionally.
- While that marinates, place the rest of the marinade in your blender. Add in honey, two tablespoons oil, and ¼ cup of cilantro. Mix until smooth, and add in pepper and salt to taste.

- Mix the peppers and onion together in a bowl and season with pepper, salt, ¼ teaspoon paprika, ½ teaspoon cumin, and two tablespoons of oil.
- Drain the marinade off the tofu. Sprinkle both sides with pepper and salt and place on the prepared baking sheet. Add the vegetables to the baking sheet next to the tofu.
- Bake for 20 to 25 minutes, stirring the veggies a couple of times until everything is tender.
- Divide the tofu and veggies among plates and top with sauce and the rest of the cilantro.
- DINNER
- ROAST BEEF AND VEGETABLES
- Serves: 6
- Ingredients:
- 1 lb red potatoes, halved

- 1 bulb fennel, thinly sliced
- 1 red onion, sliced
- Pepper
- 2 tsp rosemary, chopped
- Salt
- 2 tbsp balsamic vinegar
- 3 tbsp EVOO
- 3 lb beef rump roast, trimmed of fat
- Instructions:
- Your oven should be at 375. Brush the beef with a tablespoon of vinegar and oil. Then season with ½ teaspoon pepper, a teaspoon of rosemary, and two teaspoons of salt. Coat the potatoes, onion, and fennel with the rest of the salt, pepper, rosemary, vinegar, and oil. Place the veggies on the bottom of a nine by thirteen inch pan. Place the roast, fat side up, on the

vegetables.

- Cook until a thermometer reads 125 degrees Fahrenheit, and 1 ¼ to 1 ½ hours. Place the meat on a cutting board and rest for about ten minutes. Turn your oven up to 450. Stir the veggies and let them cook for another ten minutes. Slice the beef and serve along with the vegetables.

-
- **PHASE 3**

  - Phase 3 – low-glycemic fruit, moderate protein, moderate carb, high healthy fat

  - It sounds counter-intuitive, but healthy fats from raw seeds, olive oil, avocados, and raw nuts will trigger your body to burn the dietary fat and the stored fat. You have kept your fat intake low but flooded your body with nutrients from efficient proteins, alkalizing vegetables, and whole grains. You haven't been eating fats, and your body has been burning the stored fat for energy. You might have noticed that your clothes are fitting somewhat looser, but if your body catches on, and no dietary fats are coming in, it will start to store fat again instead of burning it.

  - Salmon helps to promote healthy hormone

balance in your adrenal and thyroid glands. Other nutrients in healthy fats will start to slow gastric emptying. This helps you feel fuller longer and stimulates the pituitary glands, and hypothalamus releases feel-good hormones and allows your body to feel satisfied and full.

- BREAKFAST
- BERRY COBBLER WITH QUINOA
- Serves: 4
- Ingredients:
- 1 c strawberries, frozen
- 2 c blackberries, frozen
- ¼ tsp cinnamon
- ¼ c almond milk
- ¼ c maple syrup
- 1 tsp vanilla
- ¼ c ground flaxseed
- ½ c coconut oil

- ½ c chopped walnuts
- ½ c quinoa flour
- ½ c cooked quinoa
- 1 c dry oats
- Instructions:
- Your oven should be at 375.
- Mix all the ingredients together, except for the berries.
- Place the berries in a nine by nine baking dish and then top with the quinoa mixture.
- Cook for 35 to 40 minutes or until it has browned. You can also serve with a drizzle of honey and a dollop of Greek yogurt.
- LUNCH
- ITALIAN TUNA SALAD
- Serves: 2
- Ingredients:
- ¼ tsp salt

- 1 tbsp lemon juice
- 1 minced garlic clove
- ¼ c chopped green olives
- ¼ c red onion, diced
- ½ sweet yellow pepper, diced
- 3-oz black olives, sliced
- ½ c parsley leaves, chopped
- 1 c diced tomatoes
- 2 cans Yellowfin Tuna in Olive oil, not drained
- Instructions:
- Place the tuna into a bowl and break up the pieces. Mix in the rest of the ingredients. You can serve on a bun or a bed of lettuce.
- DINNER
- SHEET PAN STEAK AND VEGGIES
- Serves: 6

- Ingredients:
- 2 lb top sirloin
- Pepper and salt
- 1 tsp thyme
- 3 minced garlic cloves
- 2 tbsp olive oil
- 16-oz broccoli florets
- 2 lb red potatoes
- Instructions:
- Your oven should be set to broil. Grease a baking sheet lightly.
- Parboil the potatoes for 12 to 15 minutes and drain.
- Place the broccoli and potatoes on the baking sheet. Drizzle with pepper, salt, thyme, garlic, and olive oil and toss.
- Sprinkle the steak with pepper and salt and

place on the baking sheet between the veggies.

- Broil the steak until browned, this should take about four to five minutes on each side.

-
-

-

-

-

-

-

-
- ## DOS AND DON'TS

  - Avoid these foods in all phases:
  - Fat-free "diet" foods – this includes zero-cal, fat-free, or diet foods
  - Artificial sweeteners
  - Fruit juices and dried fruit
  - Alcohol
  - Caffeine – if you have to have coffee, use organic decaffeinated
  - Refined sugars
  - Dairy
  - Corn
  - Non-sprouted wheat
  - Phase 1:
  - Meals: 3 meals and 2 fruit snacks

- Breakfast: fruit and grain, 30 minutes after waking up
- Fruit snack
- Lunch: vegetable, fruit, protein, and grain
- Fruit snack
- Dinner: vegetable, protein, and grain

- Organic when possible
- All fruits and veggies
- Protein – veggie and animal
  - Lean meat
  - Lean poultry
  - Lean fish
  - Eggs – white only
  - Beans
- Plenty or spices, herbs, broth, and condiments

- Grains
    - Sprouted and whole wheat
- Water
- No fats
- Phase 2:
- Meals
    - Breakfast: veggie and protein, 30 minutes after your get up
    - Protein snack
    - Lunch: veggie and protein
    - Protein snack
    - Dinner: veggie and protein
- Low-glycemic vegetables
- Lemon and limes
- Animal protein:
    - Lean meat

- - Lean poultry
  - Lean fish
  - Shellfish
  - Eggs- white only
- No vegetable proteins
- Condiments, spices, herbs, and broth
- No starches or grains
- No fats
- Water
- Phase 3:

- Meals

  - Breakfast: veggie, grain, protein, or fat 30 minutes after waking
  - Protein, fat, or veggie snack
  - Lunch: fruit, veggie, protein, or fat

- Protein, fat, or veggie snack
  - Dinner: starch, grain, veggie, protein, or fat

- All veggies

- Low-glycemic fruits

- Animal and veggie protein

  - Any meat
  - Liver
  - Poultry
  - Fish
  - Shellfish
  - Eggs

- Beans
- Seeds and nuts
- Non-dairy proteins

- Whole starches and grains

- Condiments, spices, herbs, and broth

- Healthy fats

- Water

-
-

-

-

-

-

-

-

-

CONCLUSION

Thank for making it through to the end of *Fast Metabolism Diet Cookbook.* Let's hope it was informative and able to provide you with all of the tools you need to achieve your goals.

Now you have plenty of recipes to get you started on your weight loss journey. You have all the information you need, and the recipes to get you started, so start today.

BOOK THREE

Cookbook For Diabetics

Who Says You Have To Give Up Your Favorite Foods?

DIANA WATSON

Table of Contents

[Introduction](#)

[Chapter 1: Diabetes And A Realistic Diet Plan](#)

[Chapter 2: Wake-Up With A Healthy Start](#)

[Chapter 3: Mid-Day Recipes](#)

- <u>Chapter 4: Dinner Time</u>

- <u>Chapter 5: Tasty Snacks</u>

- <u>Index for the Recipes</u>

- <u>Conclusion</u>

-

-

-

-

-

© Copyright 2017 by Diana Watson - All rights reserved.

The following Book is reproduced below with the goal of providing information that is as accurate and as reliable as possible. Regardless, purchasing this eBook can be seen as consent to the fact that both the publisher and the author of this book are in no way experts on the topics discussed within, and that any recommendations or suggestions made herein are for entertainment purposes only. Professionals should be consulted as needed before undertaking any of the action endorsed herein.

- This declaration is deemed fair and valid by both the American Bar Association and the Committee of Publishers Association and is legally binding throughout the United States.

- Furthermore, the transmission, duplication or reproduction of any of the following work, including precise information, will be considered an illegal act, irrespective whether it is done electronically or in print. The legality extends to creating a secondary or tertiary copy of the work or a recorded copy and is only allowed with express written consent of the Publisher. All additional rights are reserved.

- The information in the following pages is broadly considered to be a truthful and accurate account of facts, and as such any inattention, use or misuse of the information in question by the reader will render any resulting actions solely under their purview. There are no scenarios in which the publisher or the original author of this work can be in any fashion deemed liable for any hardship or damages that may befall them after undertaking information described herein.

- Additionally, the information found on the following pages is intended for informational purposes only and should thus be considered, universal. As befitting its nature, the information presented is without assurance regarding its continued validity or interim quality. Trademarks that mentioned are done without written consent and can in no way be considered an endorsement from the trademark holder.

-
-
-
-
-
-
-
-

Introduction

- This cookbook is provided and dedicated to those who have diabetes, a chronic disease which plagues over 29million individuals in the United States, alone {2014 calculations}. Out of those people, 1.7 million were 20 years or older were diagnosed with the disease in 2012.

- The following chapters will discuss some of the many choices which are available to you for a healthy breakfast, lunch, and dinner. A few healthier choices are provided for drink and snack options as well. The recipes included are healthy and relatively simple to prepare.

- You will discover how important it is to pay attention to the foods you consume on a daily basis. You have to be careful to not indulge in starches and sugars which will have an effect on your blood sugar levels.

- There are plenty of books on this subject on the market; I would personally like to thank you again for choosing this one! Every effort was made to ensure it is full of as much useful information as possible. Please enjoy!

-
- Chapter 1: Diabetes and A Realistic Diet Plan

- Suffering from the symptoms of diabetes doesn't have to be as complicated as some believe it is, if you provide a daily healthier diet outlook on the foods you consume. You can help 'ward-off' the complications with a healthy eating plan which can control your blood sugar, while at the same time help lower your risks of heart disease and cancer. These are some of the ways a healthy diet can improve your life:

- *Improves Your Overall Health*

- The amount of inflammation in your body can

be reduced with a healthy diet—as well as decreasing the triglycerides, bad cholesterol {LDL}; it also increases the good cholesterol {HDL}.

- Another diabetic complication, metabolic syndrome, is remedied with healthy carbohydrate sources in foods such as olive oil, nuts, and lean protein choices. The condition is presented with many conditions including elevated, blood sugar, blood pressure, and cholesterol which are all stressors that work as a team to cause issues including diabetes, strokes, and heart disease.

- *The Link between Strokes and Diabetes*

- For individuals who have diabetes; you are also at a greater risk for strokes and heart disease. Research provided by the American Heart Association indicates that at least 65% of the patients who have diabetes, also die from strokes and heart disease.

- This factor may be that the patients did not consume a healthy diet and often become sedentary and obese from the lack of energy and activity.

- **Components of a Health Diabetic Diet Plan**

- These are the food groups you should be most concerned with as a person with diabetes. As you will see, throughout this list and the provided recipes; you don't have to deprive yourself of the foods you enjoy. You just need to learn how to prepare and group them together. You will need to make some adjustments, but it is worth it.

- These are the food groups you should consider as part of your diabetic plan:

1. *Whole Grains*: Oats, bulgar, brown rice, barley whole grain cereals, and bread, as well as whole wheat pasta.

2. *Vegetables and fruits*

3. *Low-fat or fat-free dairy products*: Milk, cheese, and yogurt

4. *Unsaturated fats*: Nuts in moderate amounts and vegetable oils {Limit unhealthy trans fats and saturated fats, salt, and sugar}

5. *Lean Proteins:* Fish, skinless poultry, lean cuts of beef, and beans

6. These are the elements that the healthier diet will play in lowering your risk of diabetes complications:

7. *Fresh Produce*: Vegetables and fruits will provide many minerals and vitamins as well as being an excellent source of fiber. Blood glucose control and weight management are better maintained with the lower calorie content.

8. *Fiber*: Your blood sugar management, heart health, and digestion depend on fiber. The fiber can raise the sugar/glucose levels, lower the cholesterol levels, and satisfy your hunger for longer times.

9. *Low-fat Dairy:* You can acquire excellent sources of potassium which is essential to prevent the risk of osteoporosis, a thinning/weakness of the bones making them more prone to fractures. It is documented that individuals with diabetes are more likely to be at risk for these issues which make a healthier diet a reasonable step to take in the ways of

prevention.

10.

11.

12. *Lean Proteins*: Your body will be more sensitive to producing its insulin when you

13. provide the leaner choices protein. As a result, you can lower the risk of heart disease and excessive weight gain.

14. The Myths

15. Today's society is in such a churn that is sometimes difficult to realize you need a special diet until it's too late. The onset of diabetes is on the rise, but so many cases can be reversed, and some are preventable. First, and foremost, you will soon understand the essence of a good recipe guide. However, you need to dispel some of the myths involved with the disease and a diet plan. These are some of the myths about dieting and diabetes:

- *Myth #1:* Avoid sugar at all costs.

- *Fact #1:* The primary element you need to consider is to limit and properly plan the hidden sugars. Make the dessert a part of the healthy meal plan. You will notice there are several yummy choices in the recipe section.

- *Myth #2*: You will need special diabetic meals.

- *Fact #2:* Everyone eats the same foods if you are following a healthy diet—diabetic—or not. Purchasing specific foods for 'diabetics only' is essentially a waste of money {generally speaking}. After all, do you know what is packaged in the box? Many times the food has the forbidden 'hidden sugars.' Do you have time to shop and look at every ingredient on the label? Probably not.

- *Myth #3:* You have to cut way back on your carbohydrate intake.

- *Fact #3:* You need to consider the kind of carbs you are consuming; remembering the serving size is the key element. Eliminate the starchy carbs and focus on the whole grain carbs since they are digested slower and are high in fiber. It will help keep the blood sugar levels on an even kilter.

-
-
- # Chapter 2: Wake – Up With a Healthy Start
- These are just a few of the ways you can begin your day. Some of the recipe ideas can be prepared in advance. Enjoy!
- **Banana & Grapefruit**
- This delicious bowl of 'chilly' bites will surprise you!
- *Ingredients*
- 1 Tablespoon freshly chopped mint
- 1 cup sliced banana {approximately one}
- 1 {24-ounces} Jar of red grapefruit sections
- 1 Tablespoon honey
- *Directions*

1. Drain and save ¼ cup of the grapefruit juice.
2. Combine the entire batch of ingredients in a

medium serving dish.

3. Toss and serve or cover and chill.
4. Be ready in the morning, and prepare this the night before. You can even make it easily transportable.
5. *Yields*: Three {1-cup servings}

6. Oat Pancakes

7. *Ingredients*
8. 1 Cup oat flour
9. ¼ Cup artificial sweetener
10. 1 teaspoon baking powder
11. ¼ Cup rolled oats
12. 1 Tablespoon each:

- Ginger
- Cinnamon
- 1 egg/egg substitute equivalent
- ½ cup low-fat milk
- 1 teaspoon vanilla extract
- *Directions*

1. Prepare the griddle to 275ºF.
2. Combine all of the dry ingredients and then add the wet components—mixing thoroughly.
3. Cook them as a regular pancake; waiting for the bubbles to mount up before you flip them. Always check the bottom to see if it is browned to your liking before you turn the pancake over.
4. *Notes*: You can also add some blueberries which you can sprinkle on top of the batter when it is poured onto the griddle, so you don't pop them open in the mixing process. Try adding some fruit or nuts to the mixture.
5. **Rosemary Omelet and Veggies**
6. *Ingredients*
7. 2 Tbsp. Water
8. ¾ cup refrigerated egg product {Ex. Egg Beaters}
9. ¼ cup sharp cheddar cheese {shredded &

reduced-fat}

10. 1 {12-ounce} Frozen Red Potatoes {Cook-in-the-Bag}

11.   With added Green beans with rosemary butter sauce

12. Fresh chives

13. Directions

1. Prepare the veggies according to the package instructions.

2. Use some cooking spray and lightly coat a skillet—preheating it to the medium-high setting.

3. Whisk the water and egg product in a small container and pour into the prepared skillet. Let it cook undisturbed—allowing it to set. Run the spatula around the edges so that the uncooked egg will flow downward to the pan for about 30 to 60 seconds. When the mixture is set—turn off the heat.

4. Place the veggies in a nine-inch microwavable pie plate, and add the omelet to the top while folding {tucking} in the edges around the plate.
5. Sprinkle with the cheese and microwave on high {100%} power until the cheese melts, usually about thirty seconds.
6. *Note*: Green Giant Steamers brand is an excellent choice.
7. *Yields*: Three servings {One serving = 1/3 of an omelet and ½ cup of veggies}
8. *Grams of Carbs per Serving*: 18

9. Yogurt Pudding

10. *Ingredients*
11. ¼ Cup Crushed Pineapple {Can – juice pack}
12. 1 {6-ounces} Carton vanilla low-fat yogurt
13. ½ Cup fat-free milk
14. ½ Cup regular rolled oats
15. ½ teaspoon vanilla

16. 1 tablespoon flax seed meal/chia seeds
17. *Optional*:
18. Chopped red apple
19. 1/8 teaspoon toasted sliced almonds
20. *Directions*
1. Combine the pineapple, yogurt, vanilla, chia seeds, cinnamon, milk, and oats in a medium dish. Add them to a container and secure the lid.
2. Chill in the fridge for two days or at least for eight hours.
3. Stir completely, and add the almonds, if desired, as well as the apple.
4. *Yields*: Two Servings {3/4 Cup each}
5. *Grams of Carbs per Serving*: 38

6. Baked Apple

7. *Ingredients*
8. 1 Cup Fresca
9. 1 Tablespoon cornstarch

10. ¼ teaspoon cinnamon

11. 1 ½ teaspoon sweetener substitute

12. ¼ teaspoon salt

13. Apples

14. Butter for the tops of apples

15. *Directions*

1. Cut the apples in half and remove the seeds.

2. Preheat the oven to 375ºF.

3. Combine the cinnamon, salt, and cornstarch with 1 Tablespoon of Fresca.

4. Stir as you gradually add the remainder of the Fresca until it is clear and smooth.

5. Arrange the halved apples in a baking dish and empty the mixture over them while dotting each one with the butter.

6. Bake for 45 minutes to about an hour.

7. **Apple Jelly**

8. You will love the fact you know what is in your jelly when you make it from scratch. This one

is a winner!

9. *Ingredients*

10. 2 Packages unflavored gelatin

11. 4 Tablespoons artificial sweetener

12. 1-quart apple juice

13. 2 Tablespoons lemon juice

14. *Directions*

1. Mix all of the components on the list in a saucepan and blend well.

2. All you need to do is boil the jelly for about five minutes. Let it cool.

3. Pour into the containers and store in the fridge.

4.

5.

6.

7. Chapter 3: Mid-Day Recipes

8. Along about mid-day, you are probably in need of a healthy 'pick-me-up.' These are some of the ways you can get going for the rest of the day.

9. **Barbecue Ranch Wraps**

10. *Ingredients*

11. 1 -Tablespoon salad dressing/light mayonnaise

12. 2 - Tablespoons Ranch salad dressing {reduced-fat}

13. 2 Cups packaged shredded broccoli/slaw mix type

14. 4 {8-inches} Whole grain flour tortillas

15. 8 ounces cooked turkey or chicken breasts

16. 2 Tablespoons Barbecue Sauce

17. *Directions*

1. Combine the mayonnaise and ranch dressing in a medium mixing dish; blend in the broccoli.
2. Cover the tortillas with a layer of the barbecue sauce.
3. Top it off with the chicken and broccoli mixture.
4. Roll them up.
5. *Yields*: Four Servings

6. Diabetic & Heart-Healthy Stuffed Peppers

7. *Ingredients*
8. 4 Tablespoons Corn oil
9. 2 garlic cloves
10. 2 sliced onions
11. 4 diced tomatoes
12. 1 diced zucchini
13. 2 cups brown rice {cooked}
14. 4 large seeded green peppers

15. ½ cup grated cheddar cheese
16. 2 cups tomato juice
17. *Directions*
1. Set the oven in advance to 375ºF.
2. Prepare a large pan with the oil using medium heat.
3. Sauté the tomatoes, zucchini, onions, and garlic; until they are done. Add the rice and cheese to the pan.
4. Stuff the peppers with the veggie mixture and put the tops back on.
5. Empty the juice into the bottom of a casserole dish/pan and bake for 30 minutes.
6. *Yields*: Four Servings

7. Hummus and Avocado Salad Sandwiches

8. *Ingredients*
9. ½ of an avocado {peeled and sliced}
10. 1/3 Cup Mediterranean-flavor hummus

11. ¼ teaspoon black pepper
12. 1 Cup Arugula leaves
13. 4 - whole wheat, split bagel bread or sandwich thins
14. ½ Cup or {2-ounces} Gruyere cheese
15. Directions

1. Lightly grease a skillet with a small amount of cooking spray.
2. Heat the pan on the medium temperature setting or use the outdoor grill.
3. Spread some of the hummus on each of the bagel thins, and sprinkle with the pepper.
4. Begin the layer of the sandwich with the avocado slices, arugula, and shredded cheese. Place the tops on with the spread-side down, and put them on the skillet/grill.
5. Toast them for about two minutes with another object/skillet on top to keep the sandwich firm {like they use at the Waffle

House}. Flip the sandwich and cook another two minutes.

6. *Yields*: Four Servings {One sandwich}
7. *Grams of Carbs per Serving*: 26
8. **Beef and Bean Chili**
9. *Ingredients*
10. 1 Cup finely chopped onions
11. 2 Pounds ground beef
12. 2 medium carrots
13. 1 can tomato paste
14. 1 {28-ounces} Can of tomatoes – undrained and chopped
15. 1 {16-ounces} Can kidney or pinto beans
16. Chili Seasoning
17. Mild grated cheese
18. *Directions*

1. Peel and grate the carrots.
2. Prepare the beef and onions in a skillet until done, and drain the grease.

3. Combine the remainder of the ingredients with the mixture—excluding the beans.
4. Let the ingredients blend in the skillet for approximately 45 minutes, and add the beans —cooking until they are warmed.
5. Serve in a bowl with a topping of cheese.
6. Enjoy with some crackers or homemade cornbread!
7. *Yields*: 2 ½ quarts
8. **Chicken Salad with Orzo**
9. *Ingredients*
10. 1 Cup frozen/fresh corn kernels
11. 2/3 Cup dried {3-ounces} orzo pasta
12. 2 cups chopped/shredded cooked chicken breast
13. ¼ Cup Freshly cut cilantro
14. 1 Cup halved grape tomatoes
15. ½ Cup {2-ounces reduced-fat} Feta cheese
16. *Dressing:* Your choice

17. *Directions*

1. Prepare the orzo—adding the corn the last minute of the cooking time. It will cool quickly by rinsing with cold water; Drain.
2. Mix the chicken orzo mixture, cilantro, and tomatoes in a large serving bowl. Give them a sprinkle of crumbled cheese.
3. Place them in the refrigerator for a minimum of two hours—preferably 24-hours.
4. Drizzle with your favorite dressing.
5. *Yields*: Four Servings {1/4 Cup dressing and 1 Cup salad}
6. *Grams of Carbs per Serving*: 30
7. **Salmon Tacos**
8. *Ingredients*
9. 14 to 16 ounces cooked salmon
10. 1 Tbsp. Lime juice
11. 8 {6-inch} warmed tortillas
12. ½ C. thinly sliced red sweet pepper

13. 1 C. shredded cabbage with carrots
14. 1 *Sour Cream Drizzle* recipe {below}
15. Lime Wedges {*Optional*}

16. Directions

1. Gently toss the cooked salmon with the juice of the lime until saturated.
2. Add the sweet peppers, cabbage, and salmon mixture to floured tortilla.
3. Garnish each one of the tortillas with a drizzle of the sour cream or sprinkle with some cilantro, and serve with a lime wedge or two.
4. *Note:* You can substitute coleslaw mix in this recipe for the cabbage mixture.
5. *Yields*: Four Servings {2 Tacos}
6. *Grams of Carbs per Serving*: 27
7. **For the Sour Cream Drizzle:**
8. 1 Tbsp. Lime juice
9. 1 Tbsp. Fresh cilantro
10. 1/3 C. light sour cream

11. 1/8 tsp. each:
- Salt
- chili powder
- Thoroughly mix all of the listed ingredients in a mixing bowl.

Chapter 4: Dinner Time

Here are some ideas for dinner time which cover several choices:

Beef

Beef Burgundy

Ingredients

- 2 Pounds Top round steak
- ½ Cup dry - red wine
- 1 Tbsp. flour
- 1 Pouch onion soup mix {dry}
- 1 {3-ounces} Can mushrooms
- 1 ¾ - Cups water

Directions

1. Heat the oven to 350ºF.
2. Slice the steak into one-inch cubes.
3. Prepare a skillet with a small amount of vegetable spray. Add the beef and cook slowly.
4. Drain and place the meat into a 1 ½ quart casserole dish with a tight-fitting lid.
5. Combine and add the remainder of the ingredients—stirring well.
6. Cover the dish and bake for 15 additional minutes
7. You can serve over some noodles or rice. What a yummy delight!

8. Cabbage Rolls

9. *Ingredients*
10. 3 ounces ground beef
11. 1 large cabbage leaf
12. 2 minced onions
13. 1 teaspoon tomato sauce or diabetic ketchup
14. 1 tablespoon minced green pepper

15. *Directions*

1. Heat the oven to 350ºF.
2. Prepare the beef, and add the onions and green peppers for about the last five minutes.
3. Drain the ingredients and mix in the seasonings.
4. Put the components into the cabbage leaf and roll. Use a toothpick to close the leaf.
5. Bake for a short time until the cabbage leaf is cooked to the desired doneness.

6. Chipotle Meatloaf with Cilantro

7. *Ingredients*

8. 1/2 {10-ounces} Package frozen cooked brown rice – thawed—{approx. 1 ½ Cups}
9. 2/3 Cup Chipotle salsa
10. ¼ Cup frozen/refrigerated egg product {thawed}
11. 2 Tablespoons ground flax seed meal
12. 1 Lb. Ex.-lean ground beef

13. ¾ Cup chopped fresh cilantro

14. ¼ teaspoon salt

15. *Directions*

1. Set the oven temperature to 350ºF.
2. Line a baking pan with foil and cooking spray.
3. Mix the egg product, 2/3 of the salsa, salt, cilantro, and rice; lastly, add the beef and mix well.
4. Make, and place the meat mixture into a loaf pan. Bake for 40 to 45 minutes or 160ºF with a thermometer.
5. Remove the tasty meatloaf from the oven and spoon the remainder of the salsa onto the top. Let it rest for about ten minutes.
6. *Yields*: 4 {7-ounces) Servings
7. *Grams of Carbs per Serving*: 15

8. Chicken

9. Chicken Breasts & Orange Sauce

10. *Ingredients*

11. 1 ½ Pounds Chicken breasts {no bones or skin}
12. ½ teaspoon each:
- Paprika
- Tarragon
- 1 teaspoon salt
- 4 teaspoons unsaturated butter
- 1 Cup orange juice
- 1 sliced orange
- 1 Tablespoon grated orange rind
- *Directions*

1. Flavor the chicken with the pepper and salt.
2. Arrange the chicken in a casserole container and brown with the butter.
3. Add the juice, tarragon, and rind. Bake in an uncovered dish for thirty minutes.
4. Take the meal from the oven, and put the pan with the liquid/juices back in the oven. Increase the heat to thicken the sauce.

5. Enjoy the flavorsome sauce over some steamed rice or just over the chicken. Garnish with an orange slice or two.

6. Baked Chicken and Rice

7. Ingredients

8. 6 halves chicken breast {no skin}
9. 1 Package onion soup mix {divided}
10. 1 Cup cooked rice
11. 1/8 teaspoon pepper
12. 1 Can {10- ¾ ounces} Cream of mushroom soup
13. 1 ½ - Cups water

14. Directions

1. Heat the oven to 325ºF.
2. Arrange the rice on the bottom of a rectangular baking dish/pan; a 9 x 12 would work nicely.
3. Use ¼ of the soup mix, and drizzle it over the rice; add the chicken, and sprinkle the

remainder of the mix along with the pepper, water, and can of soup. Stir well.

4. Pour the soup over the breasts of chicken.

5. Cover the dish and bake for approximately two hours.

6. Chicken Cacciatora

7. *Ingredients*

8. 3 {1/2-Pounds} skinless chicken breast

9. 1 garlic clove

10. 1 tsp. oregano

11. 2 Tbsp. Olive oil

12. 1 {16-ounces} Can stewed tomatoes

13. 1 ½ C. sliced mushrooms

14. *Optional:*

- Parsley
- Pepper
- Salt
- *Directions*

1. Pour the oil in a skillet and brown the chicken

with the garlic. Give it a sprinkle of pepper, salt, and oregano before you flip it over to the other side. Discard the garlic.
2. Toss in the mushrooms until lightly browned, and pour in the tomatoes.
3. Place a top on the pan and cook for about thirty minutes, and uncover.
4. Continue to cook until the sauce is the desired consistency.
5. Top it off with some parsley.

6. Chicken Teriyaki

7. *Ingredients*
8. 1 Skinned broiler-fryer
9. 1 teaspoon each:
- Dry mustard
- Ginger
- Garlic salt
- ½ Cup Soy Sauce
- 2 Tablespoons each:

- Brown sugar substitute
- Lemon juice
- Water
- *Directions*

1. Mix together all of the ingredients—omit the chicken—in a small pan and boil.
2. Empty the contents over the chicken into a container and marinate it in the fridge for about two or more hours {a plastic baggie is excellent}.
3. You can either bake in the oven or use the grill. Use the tasty sauce for basting during the cooking process.
4. *Note: Cook in the Microwave*: 10 minutes; turn and cook ten more.
5. **Oven-Fried Chicken**
6. *Ingredients*
7. 1 Cut-up Fryer
8. ¼ cup each:

- Buttermilk
- Wheat germ
- Potato flakes
- ½ teaspoon each:
- Garlic salt
- Salt
- Paprika
- Pinch of Pepper
- *Directions*

1. Set the oven in advance to 350ºF. Lightly grease a baking dish with some cooking spray.
2. Flavor the fryer with some pepper and salt, and let it rest to blend about half an hour or more.
3. Dip it into the buttermilk. Then into this mixture—potato flakes, wheat germ, paprika, and garlic salt.
4. Arrange the chicken in the dish and bake for approximately 35 minutes.

5. Fish

6. Baby Shrimp and Mustard Tarragon Dip

7. Ingredients

8. 1 C. baby shrimp
9. 2 tsp. dried tarragon
10. 1 tsp. lemon juice
11. 1 C. mayonnaise
12. 1 ½ - tsp. white wine vinegar
13. 2 Tbsp. Dijon mustard
14. ½ cup sour cream

15. Directions

1. Combine the tarragon, mustard, vinegar, and lemon juice.
2. Blend the mayonnaise into the mixture and add the shrimp—followed by the sour cream.
3. Blend the ingredients well—cover—and chill.
4. *Yields*: Ten Servings
5. *Grams of Carbs per Serving*: 1

6. Tuna Casserole

7. Ingredients

8. 1 Can Chow Mein noodles

9. 1 Can diabetic tuna fish

10. 1 Can cream of mushroom soup

11. 1 Cup water

12. Pepper and salt

13. *Topping*: Cubes of butter

14. Directions

1. Set the temperature in the oven to 350ºF.

2. Mix all of the components.

3. Bake for one hour.

4. Have some fresh rolls to complement this tasty dish.

5. Pork

6. Saucy Thai

7. Ingredients

8. 1 {14-ounces} Package Frozen sweet pepper stir-fry vegetables

9. 1 Pound Boneless pork loin

10. ½ C. Unsweetened coconut milk {reduced-fat}

11. 3 tsp. olive oil {divided}

12. 1 1/3 C. brown rice {cooked}

13. 1 Tbsp. of Each:

- All-purpose flour
- Thai-style seasoning blend
- *Directions*

1. Thaw and drain the veggies. Trim away any fat and cut the pork into bite-size pieces; set aside.

2. Whisk the coconut milk, Thai seasoning, and flour together and set to the side.

3. In the meantime, pour one teaspoon of the oil in a pan using the medium heat setting. Toss in the veggies and cook—covered for three to five minutes until crispy but tender. When it is done; place them in a separate container.

4. Pour the remainder of the oil in the skillet and

add the pork. Cook over the med-high setting for three to five minutes. Put the vegetables back into the skillet.

5. Blend in the coconut milk mixture and continue cooking until the sauce has thickened, for one to two minutes; stir frequently.
6. Serve over a nice plate of hot cooked rice.
7. *Yields*: Four servings {1/3 cup of rice plus ¾ cup pork mixture}
8. *Grams of Carbs per Serving*: 23

9. Pork Chops and Apples

10. *Ingredients*
11. 1 medium chopped onion
12. 4 lean-cut pork chops
13. ¼ teaspoon pepper
14. 1 teaspoon pepper
15. 1 ¼ Cups Water
16. ½ teaspoon cinnamon

17. 3 Medium cooking apples

18. Directions

1. Peel and slice the apples.

2. Brown the chops and onions in a skillet.

3. Mix water, pepper along with the bouillon in a mixing dish. Add this to the skillet. Cover and let it boil.

4. Lower the heat and continue cooking for approximately twenty minutes.

5. Remove/skim away the fat and add the apples and cinnamon.

6. Cover the meal and simmer about fifteen more minutes and serve piping hot.

7. **Pork Chops and Gravy**

8. *Ingredients*

9. 1 Can cream of mushroom soup

10. 2 Tablespoons flour

11. 4 small pork chops

12. *Optional:*

- Parsley
- Pepper
- *Directions*

1. Set the oven temperature in advance to 350ºF.

2. Flavor the chops lightly with the pepper and coat them with the flour.

3. Use some cooking spray to coat a baking dish, and add the pork.

4. Empty the soup over the pork chops along with the water. {You can blend them together beforehand if you wish to make it easier.}

5. Sprinkle with the parsley {if desired}.

6. Secure the lid or use some heavy-duty foil, and bake for about 1- to 1 ½ hours.

7. Enjoy with some rice or potatoes.

8.

9. Chapter 5: Tasty Snacks
===

10. These are several items you can enjoy when you cannot resist the urge for something sweet!

11. **Applesauce Cake**

12. *Ingredients*

13. 1 Cup unsweetened applesauce

14. 2 Cups Each:

- Water
- Raisins
- 2 T. liquid sweetener
- ¾ Cup oil
- 2 eggs
- 2 Cups flour
- ¼ tsp. nutmeg
- 1 tsp. baking soda
- 1 tsp. vanilla

- *Directions*

1. Preheat the oven to 350ºF. Prepare a loaf pan with some cooking spray.
2. Add the raisins to the water and cook until the water is absorbed.
3. Put the eggs, applesauce, sweetener, and oil once the raisins are cool. Blend well.
4. Sift in the soda, nutmeg, and flour. Add the vanilla and combine.
5. Empty the batter into the baking pan and bake for approximately one hour.
6. **Banana Bread**
7. *Ingredients*
8. 4 tsp. baking powder
9. ½ Cup Splenda®
10. 1 tsp. each:

- salt
- baking powder
- 2 ½ Cups all-purpose {un-sifted}

- 1/3 Cup polyunsaturated butter
- 1 Cup mashed ripe bananas
- 2 {stiffly beaten} egg whites
- ½ Cup skim milk
- *Directions*

1. Prepare the oven setting to 350ºF. Lightly grease a loaf pan.
2. Mix the flour, Splenda, baking powder, and salt—blending well.
3. Add the milk, beaten eggs, butter, and bananas.
4. Mix using an electric mixer for one minute at the low-speed setting.
5. Pour the prepared batter into the loaf pan.
6. Place in the preheated oven for 55 to 60 minutes.
7. **Rice Pudding**
8. *Ingredients*
9. 1 Package Instant sugar-free pudding

10. 1 Cup Cooked Rice
11. 2 Cups Water
12. 1 cup of milk
13. *Optional:*

- Cinnamon

- Raisins

- *Directions*

1. Prepare the pudding by adding the above ingredients together.
2. Add the mixture to the rice, and enjoy. {Guilt-Free}

3. **Beverages**
4. **Chilly Berry**
5. You will love this tasty delight and not feel guilty!
6. *Ingredients*
7. 1 {12-ounces} Can Strawberry/Cherry carbonated beverage {sugar-free}

8. 1/3 Cup Unsweetened pineapple juice

9. ½ Cup Strawberry ice cream

10. Directions

1. Use a pretty, tall glass, add the chilled ingredients, and enjoy!

2. Garnish with a mint leaf and a sliced berry.

3. **Orange & Cream Punch**

4. Ingredients

5. 1 2/3 Cups diabetic sweetener {Splenda}

6. 1 Package unsweetened orange drink {Kool-Aid®}

7. 1/3 teaspoon vanilla {to taste}

8. Directions

1. Combine the Splenda and drink mix and add to a two-quart pitcher.

2. Add the water to the fill line and stir well. Add the vanilla, and stir again.

3. Place a lid on the pitcher and let it chill in the fridge for two to four hours. You want it super

cold.

4. Add a lemon slice and some ice; enjoy!

5. **Sparkling Fruit Drink**

6. *Ingredients*

7. 1 Quart diet ginger ale

8. Ice

9. 8 Ounces Each Unsweetened:

- Orange juice
- Grape juice
- Apple juice
- *Directions*

1. Mix the ingredients together and add the ice cubes.

2. *Yields:* Seven Servings {Nine-ounces each}

3.

4. Index for the Recipes

5. Chapter 2: Wake – Up With a Healthy Start

- Banana & Grapefruit
- Oat Pancakes
- Rosemary Omelet and Veggies
- Yogurt Pudding
- Baked Apples
- Apple Jelly

- **Chapter 3: Mid-Day Recipes**

- Barbecue Ranch Wraps
- Diabetic & Heart-Healthy Stuffed Peppers
- Hummus and Avocado Salad Sandwiches
- Beef and Bean Chili
- Chicken Salad with Orzo
- Salmon Tacos
- *For the Sour Cream Drizzle:*

- **Chapter 4: Dinner Time**
- **Beef**
- Beef Burgundy
- Cabbage Rolls
- Chipotle Meatloaf with Cilantro
- **Chicken**
- Chicken Breasts & Orange Sauce
- Baked Chicken and Rice
- Chicken Cacciatora
- Chicken Teriyaki
- Oven-Fried Chicken
- **Fish**
- Baby Shrimp and Mustard Tarragon Dip
- Tuna Casserole
- **Pork**
- Saucy Thai
- Pork Chops and Apples
- Pork Chops and Gravy

- **Chapter 5: Tasty Snacks**

- Applesauce Cake

- Banana Bread

- Rice Pudding

- **Beverages**

- Chilly Berry

- Orange & Cream Punch

- Sparkling Fruit Punch

-
-

- **Conclusion**

- Thank for viewing the *Diabetic Cookbook: Who Says You Have To Give Up Your Favorite Foods?* Let's hope it was informative and able to provide you with all of the tools you need to achieve your goals of mastering the ways you can plan a healthier meal for you and your family. The recipes provided should have given you some insight on how to proceed with your goals for diabetic healthcare management.
- The next step is to start trying out some of the healthier choices provided in this book, since they have been proven by the professionals to be beneficial to your future lifestyle changes. Don't think of it as drudgery, but as a means to live a healthy style without being hungry or

feeling deprived of your favorite foods. It is all a part of balancing your diet.

- You can do it, and you have already taken the most difficult first step; you realize you need to improve to become healthier.

-